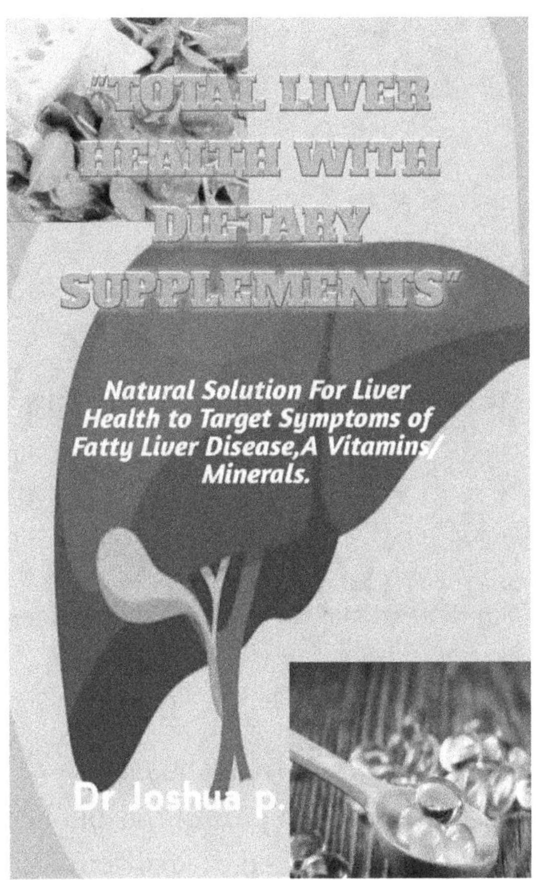

"TOTAL LIVER
HEALTH WITH
DIETARY
SUPPLEMENTS"
Natural Solution For Liver
Health to Target Symptoms of
Fatty Liver Disease, A Vitamins/
Minerals.
Dr Joshua p.

# "TOTAL LIVER HEALTH WITH DIETARY SUPPLEMENT "

*Natural Solution For Liver Health to Target Symptoms of Fatty Liver Disease, A Vitamins/Minerals.*

**Dr Joshua p.**

**Other of Dr Joshua p. books:**
HEALTHY HEART.
A COMPREHENSIVE GUIDE TO URINARY [1]TRACT HEALTH.

# Table of content

---
1

**INTRODUCTION**    5

**CHAPTER 1**    7

Why Liver Health Is Important    7

1.2 Purpose of the Dietary Liver Supplement Guide    9

**CHAPTER 2**    11

Understanding Your Liver    11

2.1 Anatomy and Function    11

2.2 Common Liver Health Issues    13

**CHAPTER 3**    17

Choosing the Right Liver Supplement    17

3.1 Essential Nutrients for Liver Health    17

3.2 Assessing the Quality of Supplements    21

3.3 Recommendations for Dosage and Use    24

To ensure the effectiveness and safety of liver supplements, it is essential to determine the proper dosage and use.    24

**CHAPTER 4**    27

Dietary Recommendations for Liver Health    27

4.1 Dietary Supplements for a Healthy Liver    28

4.3 Meal Preparation to Promote Liver Health    32

**CHAPTER 5**    35

Lifestyle practices that support the liver    35

5.1 Physical Activity and Exercise    **Error! No bookmark name given.**

5.2 Stress Management    37

5.3.Limiting alcohol consumption and smoking    39

**CHAPTER 6**    41

Recipes and meal plans,                          41

6.1 Liver-friendly Recipes                       41

6.2 Weekly Meal Schedules                        43

**CHAPTER 7**                                    47

Monitoring and tracking your progress is         47

7.1 Health Metrics to Pay Attention to     **Error!
Bookmark not defined.**

7.2 Maintaining a Liver Health Journal           50

**CHAPTER 8**                                    53

Frequently Asked Questions                       53

8.1 Frequently Asked Questions About Liver
Health                                           53

**CHAPTER 9**                                    59

References and Resources                         59

9.1 Recommended reading:                         59

9.2 Online Resources                             60

9.3 Citations and References                     61

**CHAPTER 10**                                   63

Conclusion                                       63

10.1 Key Takeaways Summary                       64

10.2 Recommendations for Preserving Liver
Health                                           66

**Table**                                        69

# INTRODUCTION

The body's chemical factory is frequently used to describe your liver, a fascinating organ.
 It is essential for processing nutrition, removing pollutants, and breaking down medications. For general health, it is crucial to maintain a healthy liver.
The liver, though, can be seriously taxed by modern lives, diets, and exposure to chemicals in the environment.

This dietary liver supplement guide is intended to assist you in appreciating the significance of liver health and to give you useful advice on how to maintain and nourish your liver with dietary supplements.

This manual will include advice on picking the appropriate supplements, adopting a diet that is friendly to the liver, and changing your lifestyle in ways that can benefit your liver health, whether you are actively trying to improve it or are treating specific difficulties.

You will have the information and resources necessary to take control of your liver health by the end of this manual and start along the path to a healthier, more active life.
 Keep in mind that having a healthy liver is essential for overall vitality, and this guide is your entry point.

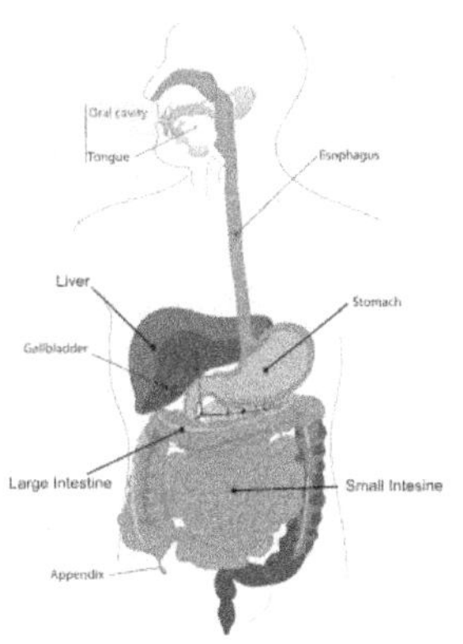

# CHAPTER 1

## Why Liver Health Is Important

One of your body's busiest organs, the liver, plays a crucial role in preserving your general health.

The following are some strong arguments in favor of making liver health a high priority:

**1. Detoxification**: Liver is in charge of filtering and expelling poisons from your bloodstream. It aids in the removal of damaging toxins from your body, preventing their buildup and negative effects.

**2. Metabolism**: The liver is essential for metabolizing a variety of foods, including lipids, proteins, and carbs. It is essential to the creation of energy and the utilization of nutrients.

**3. Nutrient Storage:** The liver stores vital nutrients, such as vitamins and minerals, and releases them as needed.

**4. Blood Sugar Control**: By storing and releasing glucose when necessary, it contributes to the stability of blood sugar levels.

**5. Digestive System:** The digestive system needs bile, which is produced by the liver, to break down lipids.
This promotes effective nutrient absorption and digestion.

**6. Support for the immune system:** The liver aids in the immune system's ability to fight off illnesses and infections.

**7.Blood Clotting:** It generates the blood clotting proteins needed to stop excessive bleeding from wounds.

8. Controlling cholesterol levels is vital for heart health and is something the liver helps with.
Your liver is essentially a multitasking powerhouse, and its condition has an impact on your general health.

Your body works best when your liver is in good shape.

## 1.2 Purpose of the Dietary Liver Supplement Guide

This Dietary Liver Supplement Guide's main goal is to arm you with the information and helpful advice you need to choose dietary liver supplements wisely.

The following goals are specifically addressed in this guide:

1. **Educate and Inform:** We will provide you with a thorough grasp of dietary liver supplements, including their advantages, possible drawbacks, and how they can be a beneficial addition to your health regimen.

2. **Selection and usage recommendations:** You'll discover how to select the ideal dietary liver supplements depending on your unique requirements and situation.

On dose, application, and probable drug interactions, we'll provide advice.

**3. Encourage liver health:** This manual will assist you in adopting a lifestyle that supports the health of your liver by providing information on diet, exercise, and stress reduction methods.

**4. Encourage informed decisions:** We want you to have faith in the choices you make regarding your liver's health.
 You will be prepared to make decisions that are good for your liver and general health by the end of this book.

**5. "A Path to Vitality"** This guide's main goal is to help you embark on a path towards greater health and energy by concentrating on the health of your liver.
This manual is your travel companion as you work towards a healthier, more energetic existence because your liver is the foundation of your general health.

# CHAPTER 2

## Understanding Your Liver

Understanding the anatomy and function of your liver, a critical and complicated organ, is the first step in recognising its importance in preserving your general health.

# 2.1 Anatomy and Function

The largest internal organ in your body, the liver, is situated on the upper right side of your belly, directly below the diaphragm.
It is segmented into multiple lobes and has a recognisable wedge-like form. Here is a closer look at its structure and main operations:

## Anatomy:

• **Hepatocytes:** These are the main metabolic cells in the liver and are in charge of several metabolic processes.

• **Bile Ducts**: Bile, which is made by the liver, is crucial for the digestion of fats.
Through a network of bile ducts, bile is carried from the liver to the gallbladder and the small intestine.

• **Blood Supply**: A dual blood supply is provided to the liver.
Blood that is rich in nutrients and low in oxygen enters the body through the portal vein.

• **Gallbladder:** The liver produces bile, which the gallbladder stores and releases into the small intestine when digestion calls for it.

## Key function :

1. **Detoxification:** The liver processes and removes toxins from the blood, making them less toxic and prepared for excretion.

2. **Metabolism:** To produce energy and necessary molecules, it metabolizes substances like carbs, proteins, and lipids.

**3. Bile Production:** Bile, which is created by the liver, is necessary for breaking down dietary lipids.

**4. Nutrient Storage:** When your body requires them, it releases stored nutrients like vitamins and glycogen.

**5. Blood Sugar Regulation:** The liver controls blood sugar levels by storing or releasing glucose.

**6. Protein Synthesis:** It produces proteins that are essential for nutrition transport, immunological function, and blood coagulation.

**7. Immune support** By eliminating bacteria and other foreign substances from the blood, the liver contributes to the immunological response.

## 2.2 Common Liver Health Issues

Despite being a tough organ, the liver is susceptible to a number of health problems because of a number of factors, including genetics, way of life, and environmental effects. It is crucial to comprehend these typical liver health issues in order to identify prospective problems and take preventative measures to keep the liver healthy.

Here are a few typical issues with the health of the liver:

**1. Fatty Liver Disease:** Fatty Liver Disease is characterized by a buildup of fat in liver cells and may be brought on by obesity, a poor diet, excessive alcohol consumption, or other medical disorders.

Modern culture is increasingly concerned about non-alcoholic fatty liver disease (NAFLD), which can develop into more serious forms like non-alcoholic steatohepatitis (NASH).

**2. Hepatitis :** Hepatitis is an inflammation of the liver frequently brought on by viral infections (such as hepatitis A, B, or C).

If left untreated, it can cause symptoms like jaundice, exhaustion, and liver damage.

**3. Cirrhosis**:Cirrhosis is the advanced stage of the liver's scarring (fibrosis), which is brought on by sustained liver injury.

It can be brought on by hepatitis, prolonged alcoholism, or other health issues. Liver failure may result from cirrhosis.

**4. Hepatocellular carcinoma** (HCC), a primary liver cancer, can arise inside the liver. Furthermore, cancer from other regions of the body may metastasize to the liver.

**5. Liver Fibrosis:** The development of scar tissue in the liver is known as fibrosis.

It frequently develops from ongoing liver inflammation and can be a prelude to cirrhosis.

**6. Alcohol-Related Liver Disease:** Chronic alcohol use can harm the liver, resulting in cirrhosis in the end as well as alcoholic fatty liver disease and alcoholic hepatitis.

7. Autoimmune liver conditions Autoimmune diseases that affect the liver and bile ducts include autoimmune hepatitis, primary biliary

cholangitis, and primary sclerosing cholangitis.

**8. Wilson's illness:** This rare hereditary condition causes aberrant copper accumulation in the liver and other tissues.

**9. Hemochromatosis:** This genetic disorder causes the body to absorb excessive amounts of iron, which overburdens the liver and other organs with iron.

**10. Toxic liver damage**: acute or chronic liver injury can result from exposure to specific drugs, chemicals, or poisons.

It is essential to recognise the warning signs and symptoms of these liver health problems and to take the proper preventative and therapeutic measures.
You will gain useful knowledge and suggestions on how to support your liver and keep it functioning at its best from this manual.

# CHAPTER 3

## Choosing the Right Liver Supplement

Making the right liver supplement choice is essential to maintaining the health of your liver.

Making educated decisions on liver supplements will be made easier for you thanks to this section's explanation of the crucial nutrients that contribute to liver health.

## 3.1 Essential Nutrients for Liver Health

To perform at its best and keep itself healthy, your liver needs a variety of crucial nutrients. These vitamins and minerals can be obtained either naturally or through supplementation.

The following are some essential nutrients that are good for liver health:

1. **Antioxidants:** Antioxidants, including vitamins C, E, and selenium, help shield the liver from oxidative stress and harm brought on by free radicals.

2. **B vitamins:** The liver's different metabolic functions depend on B vitamins, including B1 (thiamine), B2 (riboflavin), B3 (niacin), B6 (pyridoxine), B9 (folate), and B12 (cobalamin).

3. **Vitamin D :**Vitamin D helps to control liver illnesses and plays a part in lowering liver inflammation.

4 **Vitamin K:** A lack of this vitamin might cause bleeding issues as it is essential for healthy blood coagulation.

**5. Required Amino Acids:** Methionine and cysteine are essential amino acids for the production of glutathione, a strong antioxidant that aids liver detoxification.

**6. Materials:** Zinc and magnesium are minerals that support the general health of the liver and are involved in the detoxification processes of the liver.

**7. Omega-3 Fatty Acids:** Due to their anti-inflammatory qualities, these beneficial fats can help lessen liver inflammation and improve liver health.

**8. Silymarin,** or milk thistle An herbal supplement that has been investigated for its capacity to support liver regeneration and protect liver cells

**9. Curcumin,** or turmeric Curcumin, which is well-known for its anti-inflammatory and antioxidant qualities, might be useful for treating liver disorders.

**10.N-acetyl cysteine (NAC):** This derivative of an amino acid serves as a building block for glutathione, a vital liver antioxidant.

It's important to speak with a doctor before beginning any liver supplement regimen, especially if you have a pre-existing liver ailment or are using other medications.
They can advise you on the precise vitamins and amounts that are best for your particular diet.

## 3.2 Assessing the Quality of Supplements

It's critical to evaluate the quality of liver supplements while making your selection to make sure you're getting secure, useful products.

When assessing the quality of supplements, keep the following points in mind:

**1.Brand Reputation**: Choose well-known, trustworthy manufacturers that have a track record of creating top-notch supplements. Examine the reputation and client feedback of the manufacturer.

**2. Third-party evaluation**: Look for supplements that have been quality and purity tested by a third party.

A good sign of quality can be a certification from a company in the U.S. Pharmacopoeia (USP) or NSF International.

**3. Components:** Pay close attention to the ingredient list. In order to boost liver health, make sure the supplement has the particular nutrients or substances you're seeking.

4 Dosage and Concentration Verify the supplement's active component dose.
It needs to correspond to your particular requirements and any advice given by your healthcare practitioner.

**5. The Supplement's Format:** If the supplement is a pill, capsule, liquid, or powder, take it into consideration. Pick a form that is simple for you to complete and handy for you.

**6. Ingredients and Fillers:** Avoid supplements that contain fake chemicals, fillers, or needless additives.

It is best to have a simple, short list of ingredients.

**7. Expiration Date:** Verify the supplement's expiration date and that it hasn't passed its expiration date.

8. Information on allergens Check the supplement for any potential allergens like gluten, soy, or dairy if you have allergies or sensitivities.

# 3.3 Recommendations for Dosage and Use

To ensure the effectiveness and safety of liver supplements, it is essential to determine the proper dosage and use.

Before beginning any supplement regimen, it is imperative to speak with a healthcare expert because every person has different needs. Here are some broad guidelines for dosing and application:

**1. Consult a healthcare professional first**: Before beginning any liver supplement, seek the advice of a healthcare professional, such as a doctor or qualified dietitian.

They can evaluate your individual health requirements and suggest the best supplements and dosages for you.

**2. Follow Recommended Dosages**: Comply with the suggested dosages shown on the label of the supplement or as directed by your healthcare provider.

Certain nutrients might be dangerous if taken in excess.

**3. Continuity:** Use the supplement as prescribed consistently.

Since liver health frequently improves gradually, it's crucial to follow the programme.

**4. Scheduling and Directions**: Any particular directions for when and how to take the supplement should be followed.

Others work better on an empty stomach, while some may be more effective when taken with food.

**5. Watch for negative effects**: Be careful of any negative consequences.

Consult your healthcare professional and stop taking the supplement if you encounter any strange symptoms.

**6. Potential Interactions**: Let your doctor know if you're taking any other drugs or dietary supplements.

Some dietary supplements and medicines may interact, perhaps reducing the efficacy or safety of both.

Keep in mind that supplements are supposed to support a healthy lifestyle and diet.

They shouldn't be used as an alternative to a balanced diet.

To properly support the health of your liver, your healthcare professional can assist you in developing a comprehensive plan that may include supplements.

# CHAPTER 4

## Dietary Recommendations for Liver Health

Making informed dietary decisions is essential for promoting liver health.

In order to support liver health, this section offers guidance on the kinds of foods that can be beneficial to your liver, lists of foods to limit or avoid, and advice on how to plan meals.

# 4.1 Dietary Supplements for a Healthy Liver

Certain meals can actively support the health of the liver.

Including these in your diet can support and improve the function of your liver.

**1.Start with leafy greens**: Antioxidants and chlorophyll are abundant in foods including spinach, kale, and rocket, which support liver detoxification.

**2. "cruciferous vegetable"** compounds in cauliflower, broccoli, and Brussels sprouts aid liver detoxification procedures.

**3. Fruits:** Apples, berries, and citrus fruits all include antioxidants and vitamin C, which help to lessen liver inflammation.

**4. Gladiator**: Allicin, a substance found in garlic, aids liver detoxification and may aid in lowering liver fat.

**5. Turmeric** : The primary ingredient in turmeric, curcumin, has anti-inflammatory and antioxidant qualities that are advantageous to the liver.

**6. Nuts and seeds**: almonds, walnuts, and flaxseeds are excellent sources of the antioxidants and good fats that support the health of the liver.

7 **"Fatty Fish"** Omega-3 fatty acids, which are abundant in salmon, mackerel, and sardines, help to prevent liver inflammation.

**8 Green Tea**: Catechins, which are antioxidants that support liver function, are abundant in green tea.

**9. Complete Grains**: Foods like oats and brown rice offer fiber and minerals that help keep blood sugar levels constant.

**10**. Lean proteins To ease the strain on the liver, choose lean protein sources like fish, chicken, and turkey.

## 4.2 Foods to Steer Clear of:

Some foods should be avoided or consumed in moderation as they can stress the liver.

**1. Processed foods**: These foods can cause inflammation and fatty liver disease by being high in sugar and sodium.

**2. Sugary Beverages**: Sugar-heavy beverages like soda and excessive fruit juices can be harmful to the liver's health.

**3. Abuse of alcohol** : A well-known liver toxin is alcohol. For the best liver health, cut back on or completely avoid alcohol usage.

**4. Fried and quick meals**: These frequently include large amounts of harmful fats, which can cause liver fat to build up.

**5. Too much salt**: Consuming too much salt can cause liver inflammation and fluid retention. Pay attention to how much salt is in your diet.

**6. Trans Fats**: Trans fats, which are present in several processed foods and margarines, might raise liver fat and inflammation.

**7. Meats that are red and processed** :Red and processed meat overconsumption may be a factor in liver problems.

Pick lean cuts and control how much you eat.

# 4.3 Meal Preparation to Promote Liver Health

Planning your meals is a smart strategy to guarantee that you regularly support your liver.

When designing liver-friendly menus, keep the following in mind:

**1.**Make sure your diet includes a variety of fruits, vegetables, lean proteins, and healthy grains.

Watch your portion sizes to keep your weight in check, which will relieve some of the strain on your liver.

**2.**Drink plenty of water throughout the day to stay hydrated.
Limit or abstain from alcohol use.

Reduce frying while increasing healthy cooking techniques like baking, steaming, or grilling.

Create nutritious and sustaining snacks and meals that are balanced.

**3**.A diet that supports liver health is not only good for your liver but also for your general health.

You may improve your quality of life and maintain a healthy liver by following these dietary recommendations.

# CHAPTER 5

## Lifestyle practices that support the liver

Along with a balanced diet, some lifestyle choices are essential for maintaining the health of your liver.

This section sheds light on the significance of exercise, stress reduction, and moderation in alcohol and tobacco use for general liver health.

# 5.1 Physical Activity and Exercise

The key to preserving a healthy liver and general wellbeing is regular exercise. Here are some reasons why exercise is good for your liver:

**1. Weight Control**: Exercise aids in weight management and lowers the risk of obesity-related non-alcoholic fatty liver disease (NAFLD).

**2 .Insulin Sensitivity**: Exercise improves insulin sensitivity, which lowers the risk of type 2 diabetes and the associated liver problems.

**3. Reduction of Fat**: Exercise can enhance liver function and lower liver fat levels.

**4. Detoxification:** Exercise-induced sweating can assist the body's detoxification process and lighten the burden on the liver.

Aim for at least 150 minutes of moderately intense cardiovascular exercise or 75 minutes of vigorously intense aerobic exercise each week, along with muscle-strengthening exercises on two or more days each week, to support your liver.

## 5.2 Stress Management

In addition to improving your mental health, stress management is also good for your liver. Stress that is constant might cause bad behaviors and liver issues.

**Here are some benefits of stress management**:

**1. Healthy Lifestyle Decisions**: The chance of using harmful coping strategies, such as binge eating or excessive alcohol intake, can be decreased by managing stress.

**2. Reduction of Inflammation:**Techniques for stress reduction like meditation and relaxation can aid in lowering inflammation, which is bad for the liver.

**3.**Hormones that are in balance Hormones like cortisol, when raised for long periods of time, can have a deleterious impact on liver function as a result of chronic stress.

**4.** Put stress-reduction practices first to support the health of your liver and body as a whole.
Examples include mindfulness, yoga, deep breathing exercises, and relaxation techniques.

# 5.3.Limiting alcohol consumption and smoking

Excessive alcohol use and smoking are two of the most important things that might damage your liver.

**1.Drinking alcohol**: The liver is in charge of digesting alcoholic beverages.

Alcoholic liver disease, such as fatty liver, alcoholic hepatitis, and cirrhosis, can result from excessive consumption.

You should control your alcohol consumption and, if required, seek expert assistance.

**2.Smoking**: Your liver is exposed to hazardous chemicals when you smoke. Additionally, it might make liver cancer more likely.

One of the best things you can do for the health of your liver is to stop smoking.

You may greatly lessen the stress on your liver and support its health by cutting down on or ending your alcohol usage and smoking.

By incorporating these lifestyle practices into your everyday routine, you may promote the health of your liver and improve your general quality of life.
Given the importance of the liver to your overall health, caring for it is essential.

# CHAPTER 6

## Recipes and meal plans,

A great way to promote the health of your liver is to develop recipes and meal plans that are liver-friendly. We'll give you some wholesome recipes and illustrative weekly meal plans in this area to help you support the health of your liver.

## 6.1 Liver-friendly Recipes

**Here are a few dishes that contain nutrients that support the liver:**

**Green Smoothie That's Safe for Your Liver**

Ingredients: 1/2 cucumber, 1 green apple, and 1 cup of spinach or kale.1 cup of water or coconut water; 1/8-inch slice of fresh ginger; 1/2 lemon (juiced)

1. Blend each item until it is completely smooth.

Salmon with lemon and turmeric

Ingredients: 2 filets of salmon1 teaspoon of turmeric powder1 lemon (zested and juiced), 2 garlic cloves, and 1 tablespoon of olive oilTo taste, salt and pepper

Instructions:1. Combine the turmeric, garlic, lemon zest, olive oil, salt, and pepper in a bowl.2. Rub the salmon filets with the mixture.

3.Sprinkle the fish with lemon juice.4. Grill or bake the salmon until it is fully done.

## Stir-fry with Quinoa and Vegetables

1 cup of quinoa, 2 cups of water or vegetable broth, 2 cups of mixed veggies (such as broccoli, bell peppers,

and snap peas), and 2 tablespoons of low-sodium soy sauce are the ingredients.

1 teaspoon sesame oil1 minced clove of garlic

Instructions:1. Prepare the quinoa as directed on the package, either in water or vegetable broth.

2.Stir-fry mixed vegetables in a sizable skillet with sesame oil, soy sauce, and garlic.

3.

Top quinoa with stir-fried vegetables.

# 6.2 Weekly Meal Schedules

Here is a typical menu for a week that promotes liver health:

**Day 1**: Green smoothie for the liver for breakfast; grilled chicken salad with leafy greens and citrus dressing for lunch; and baked salmon with roasted asparagus and quinoa for dinner.

**Day 2:**Greek yogurt with berries and honey for breakfast Quinoa and vegetables are stir-fried for lunch.

Dinner will be lentil soup and steamed broccoli.

**Day 3**: For breakfast, have muesli with cinnamon and sliced apples.

Tuna salad on whole-grain toast for lunch; grilled turkey breast with sautéed spinach and sweet potatoes for dinner.

**Day 4:** Eggs scrambled with spinach and tomatoes for breakfastBrown rice and black bean bowl for lunch with salsa and avocadoFor dinner, steamed green beans were served with baked cod with lemon and herbs.

**Day 5:** Banana slices on whole-grain bread with almond butter for breakfastQuinoa salad with cucumber, lemon, and chickpeas for lunch Dressing with TahiniBrown rice with stir-fried tofu and mixed vegetables for dinner

**Day 6:** Breakfast smoothie made with Greek yogurt, berries, kale, and a scoop of flaxseedsFor lunch, a chicken breast filled with spinach and feta is served with roasted Brussels sprouts.

For supper, prepare grilled prawns with quinoa and a mango salsa.

**Day 7:** Chia seed pudding for breakfast with sliced strawberries and almondsLunch: whole-grain crackers and spinach and lentil soup.

Dinner will consist of roasted chicken breast, mashed cauliflower, and steamed carrots.

These are merely examples of meal plans that you can modify to suit your tastes and dietary requirements.

Make sure to seek individualized guidance on meal planning for liver health from a healthcare professional or trained dietitian

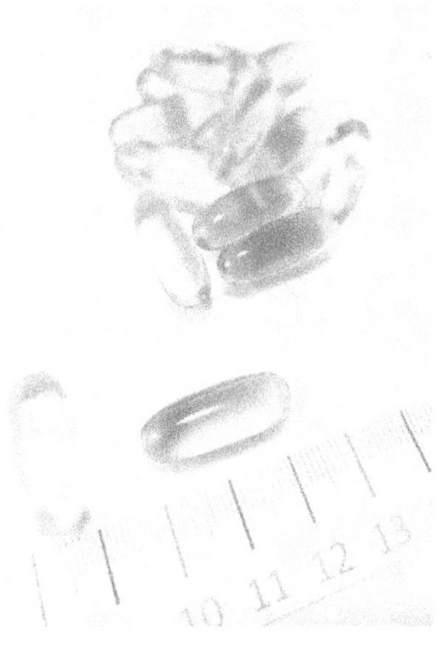

# CHAPTER 7

## Monitoring and tracking your progress is

Making wise decisions and modifications requires keeping a close eye on your liver health and tracking your progress.

This section discusses the health indicators you should pay attention to and the advantages of keeping a liver health notebook.

## 7.1 Health Metrics to Pay Attention to

Monitoring particular health indicators can give you information about the condition of your liver and your general health.

Think about monitoring the following:

**1. Liver function assessments:** These blood tests, which check for liver enzyme levels, include ALT (alanine transaminase) and AST (aspartate transaminase). Elevated levels could be a sign of inflammation or injury to the liver.

**2. Complete Blood Count:** Red and white blood cell counts, which can give hints about liver health, are part of the CBC, which evaluates your general health.

**3. Liver Imaging:** Imaging examinations such as ultrasounds, CT scans, or MRIs can identify the size, shape, and any abnormalities of the liver.

**4. Body Mass Index (BMI):** The ratio of your weight to your height can be used to determine your level of obesity, which is a risk factor for fatty liver disease.

**5. Blood Sugar Levels**: Blood sugar levels can be monitored on a regular basis to monitor diabetes risk and liver damage.

**6. Cholesterol Concentrations**: High cholesterol levels can raise the risk of cardiovascular problems and fatty liver disease.

**7. Blood pressure**: Monitoring your statistics is essential since liver problems can be exacerbated by elevated blood pressure.

**8. Drinking Alcohol**: Keep track of your alcohol consumption to make sure it stays within the advised ranges.

**9. Smoking Customs:** Monitoring your smoking patterns and making an effort to stop will greatly improve liver health.

## 7.2 Maintaining a Liver Health Journal

Keeping a liver health journal can be a very helpful tool for improving your liver health. How to make and use one is shown below.

**1. Record Your Diet**: List the items, serving amounts, and meal times you consume. Any liver-supporting supplements you are taking should be noted.

**2. Physical Exercise:** Keep a journal of your workouts, noting the time spent and the level of difficulty.

Liver health is supported by regular physical activity.

**3. Reactions and Symptoms**: Any unexpected signs or reactions, whether they have to do with your liver or your general health, should be noted.

You can use this to spot trends and potential triggers.

**4.** List all of the prescription drugs and dietary supplements you are using, along with their dosage and frequency.

**5. Alcohol and Smoking**: If applicable, list your alcohol intake and smoking patterns.

**6. Stress levels**: Consider your everyday stress levels and any stress-reduction strategies you may be employing.

**7. Health Measures:** Keep an eye on the health measures listed in Section and make note of any adjustments or trends.

**8.** Set concrete objectives to enhance the health of your liver and track your progress in achieving these objectives.

By keeping a liver health journal, you may see trends and choose your lifestyle, diet, and supplements with knowledge.

It's a useful tool for collaborating closely with medical experts to improve the condition of your liver.

# CHAPTER 8

## Frequently Asked Questions

This section responds to some often-asked questions and worries about liver health.

You're not the only one who worries about the health of your liver.

These frequently asked questions are addressed below:

## 8.1 Frequently Asked Questions About Liver Health

**Q1.What are typical indications of liver issues?**

**Q1.** Symptoms of liver problems include jaundice, or a yellowing of the skin and eyes; lethargy; unexplained weight loss; stomach pain; dark urine; pale feces; and swelling in the belly and legs.

Regular checkups are crucial since early-stage liver issues can be asymptomatic.

**Q2: Is it possible to undo liver damage?**

A2: The liver is a tough organ with a remarkable capacity for regeneration.

With certain lifestyle adjustments, such as following a balanced diet, using less alcohol, and getting to a healthy weight, liver damage may be able to be reversed.

Advanced liver disease, however, can call for medical treatment or a liver transplant.

## Q3.How can I avoid developing fatty liver disease?

A3: Maintaining a healthy weight, eating a balanced diet high in fruits, vegetables, and whole grains, and exercising frequently are frequently associated with preventing fatty liver disease.

It's also crucial to control underlying diseases like diabetes and reduce or stop drinking alcohol.

## Q4: Is it safe to take liver supplements?

A4: When taken properly, liver supplements can be safe, but you should always talk to your doctor before beginning any supplement regimen.

Based on your unique requirements and medical conditions, they can advise you on the best vitamins and quantities.

## Q5.How can I lower my risk of developing liver cancer?

A5: A combination of good lifestyle choices, such as hepatitis B and C vaccinations, maintaining a healthy weight, limiting alcohol use, and refraining from high-risk behaviors like sharing needles, can lower the risk of liver cancer.

## Q6.What constitutes a wholesome diet for liver health?

A6: A diet rich in fruits, vegetables, whole grains, lean proteins, and healthy fats like those found in fish and nuts promotes liver health.

It's also crucial to cut back on processed meals, sugar, and salt. Balance and moderation are essential.

**Q7.Can someone with a liver illness lead a normal life?**

A7: Many people with liver illnesses can live fulfilling and normal lives if they are appropriately controlled.

Effective management and early diagnosis are essential.

To get advice, speak with medical professionals.

**Q8. Can someone who has a fatty liver consume alcohol?**

A8: It's generally advised to stay away from alcohol if you have a fatty liver because it can make things worse.

It's recommended to avoid alcohol or adhere to your doctor's recommendations if you have a fatty liver or any other liver issue.

**Q9. How frequently should my liver be examined?**

A9: Your risk factors and general health determine how frequently you should have your liver checked.

An annual checkup with routine liver function tests is sufficient for many people. For specific advice, though, speak with your healthcare professional.

These responses offer broad advice, but it's vital to speak with a healthcare provider who can take into account your particular circumstances for personalized advice and to address certain health problems.

# CHAPTER 9

## References and Resources

Here are some suggested readings, websites, and references that you might check out in your quest to learn more about liver health and how to support it:

## 9.1 Recommended reading:

1. Michelle Lai's "Liver Healing Diet"
2. Anthony William's "Liver Rescue"

## 9.2 Online Resources

1.    [American Liver Foundation] (https://www.liverfoundation.org/):    A useful resource for knowledge on the health of the liver, conditions that affect it, and assistance.

2. The National Institute of Diabetes and Digestive and Kidney Diseases (NIDDK) provides information and resources on the health of the liver and liver illnesses.

3.    [Mayo Clinic: Liver Disease] (https://www.mayoclinic.org/diseases-conditions/liver-disease/symptoms-causes/syc-20374502):    Offers in-depth information on liver health and problems that are connected.

4.      [WebMD: Liver Health] (https://www.webmd.com/hepatitis/ss/sli deshow-liver-overview): A selection of articles and slideshows on matters relating to the liver and its health

5. [MedlinePlus: Liver Diseases]: This National Library of Medicine website provides information on liver diseases.

# 9.3 Citations and References

On our research if you find help do recommend us to others let's save lives together, and also , you can discover scientific and medical references about liver health in respected medical magazines like:

1. The American Association for the Study of Liver Diseases' magazine "Hepatology"

2. The European Association for the Study of the Liver's journal, "Liver International"

3. The European Association for the Study of the Liver's periodical "Journal of Hepatology"

4. The American Gastroenterological Association's magazine "Gastroenterology"5. The medical publication "World Journal of Gastroenterology" is open-access.

Many academic institutes, hospitals, and governmental health organizations also carry out research and offer comprehensive information regarding liver health and disorders related to the liver.

For specific references, look up research papers and studies on liver health and specific liver disorders in scholarly databases like PubMed or Google Scholar.

These sites can give you in-depth, current information to help you learn more.

# CHAPTER 10

## Conclusion

Thanks for reading this Dietary Liver Supplement Guide, and best of luck! We've discussed a variety of subjects connected to liver health, dietary liver supplements, and lifestyle decisions that might promote the health of your liver.

We will highlight the most important points in this final section and provide motivation for sustaining liver health.

# 10.1 Key Takeaways Summary

You've learned more about several facets of liver health throughout this guide:

**Knowing Your Liver**: We looked at the liver's anatomy and functioning, highlighting how important it is to your general health.

**Common liver health problems include**: The first step in treating common liver issues is recognising them.
Hepatitis, cirrhosis, fatty liver disease, and other topics were covered.

**Choosing the Right Liver Supplement**: Knowledge of supplement quality assessment and dosage calculations is essential for making well-informed decisions.

**Dietary Recommendations for Liver Health:** Whole foods, lean proteins, lots of fruits and vegetables, and a moderate intake of fats, sugar, and salt are all components of a diet that is beneficial to the liver.

Lifestyle Practices for Supporting the Liver For optimum liver health, we emphasized the value of exercise, stress reduction, and moderation in alcohol and tobacco use.

**Recipes and meal suggestions:** To assist you in making better dietary decisions, we have offered sample meal plans and dishes that are kind to the liver.

**Tracking Your Progress and Monitoring It:** You can follow your path towards better liver health by monitoring your health indicators and keeping a liver health notebook.

Frequently Asked Questions We addressed some of your worries by responding to frequent questions concerning liver health.

Resources and references include suggestions for more reading, links to internet sources, and references so you may carry out more study.

# 10.2 Recommendations for Preserving Liver Health

An amazing organ with a remarkable capacity for regeneration is your liver.
It's never too late to begin improving your liver care.

You can support your liver in its crucial duties and maintain your general wellbeing by adhering to the recommendations provided in this handbook, choosing a healthy lifestyle, and remaining informed.

Keep in mind that even tiny adjustments can have a big impact on liver health.

Your dedication to liver health is an essential step in your journey towards better health, regardless of whether you're trying to avoid liver issues, manage an existing ailment, or simply improve your general wellbeing.

Consult a healthcare professional if you have any specific questions or concerns regarding the condition of your liver.

They may offer tailored advice and make sure that your strategy fits your particular demands.

We appreciate you taking the time to read more about liver health and dietary liver supplements.
Taking care of your liver is a meaningful act of self-care and well-being because your health is a priceless possession.

# Table

| Day 1 | Medication | Results |
|---|---|---|
| Day 2 | | |

| Day 3 | | |
| --- | --- | --- |
| Day 4 | | |
| Day 5 | | |

| Day 6 | | |
| Day 7 | | |
| Day 8 | | |
| Day 9 | | |

| Day 10 | | |
| Day 11 | | |
| | | |
| Day 12 | | |

| Day 13 | | |
| --- | --- | --- |
| Day 14 | | |
| Day 15 | | |

| Day 16 | | |
| --- | --- | --- |
| Day 17 | | |
| Day 18 | | |

Day 19

Day 20

Day 21

| Day 22 | | |
| --- | --- | --- |
| Day 23 | | |
| Day 24 | | |

| Day 25 | | |
| --- | --- | --- |
| Day 26 | | |
| Day 27 | | |
| Day 28 | | |

| Day 29 | | |
| --- | --- | --- |

www.ingramcontent.com/pod-product-compliance
Lightning Source LLC
Chambersburg PA
CBHW061006260726

48661CB00005B/2079